Health Care Reform and Child Welfare

Meeting the Needs of Abused and Neglected Children

by Madelyn DeWoody

Child Welfare League of America
Washington, DC

CHILD WELFARE LEAGUE OF AMERICA, INC.
440 First Street, NW, Suite 310, Washington, DC 20001-2085

CURRENT PRINTING (last digit)
10 9 8 7 6 5 4 3 2 1

Cover and text design by Deborah Finette

Printed in the United States of America

ISBN # 0–87868–507–3

CONTENTS

PREFACE

As the health care reform debate continues to unfold, we can expect to see a growing number of proposals directed at changing the American health care system. Up to now, many proposals have been advanced but none has addressed specifically the health care needs of the children and youths served by the child welfare system. Advocates for vulnerable children and youths must be able to clearly illustrate the full range of health care needs associated with child abuse and neglect if they are to educate legislators and policymakers about how the health care system can best meet the needs of these children and youths.

This document represents the best efforts of the Child Welfare League of America to define the range of health care services needed by children and youths in the child welfare system—services that *should* be included in the benefit package of any health care proposal. I want to thank Madelyn DeWoody for taking the lead in developing, researching, and writing this document; Ilisa Halpern for her excellent research; Nickola Dixon for her invaluable word processing skills; and Eve Malakoff-Klein for editing and finalizing this document. We hope that the information presented here will assist child advocates in their efforts to make positive changes in our health care system in behalf of our country's most vulnerable children, youths, and families. We also hope that this document will be helpful to policymakers at the state and federal levels as they continue to look seriously at the much-needed reform of America's health care system.

David S. Liederman
Executive Director
Child Welfare League of America

The Health Status of Children and Youths in the Child Welfare System

In 1992, child welfare agencies received almost three million reports of child abuse and neglect.[1] Between 35 and 50 percent of these referrals resulted in a finding of abuse or neglect.[2] In the same year, 45 out of every 1,000 children in the United States were victims of child abuse and neglect. That figure is 7 percent higher than the number reported in 1991 and 50 percent higher than the number reported in 1985.[3]

Health concerns are inevitably linked with child abuse and neglect. In many instances, the abuse or neglect itself is health related. Parental drug and alcohol abuse, infection from the Human Immunodeficiency Virus (HIV), and medical and debilitating conditions may set the stage for situations in which abuse or neglect is likely to occur. At the same time, abuse and neglect place children and youths at particular risk of physical, mental health, and developmental problems. Because of these factors, children and youths in the child welfare system and their caregivers need primary health care services, specialized medical and health care services, mental health services, alcohol and other drug abuse prevention and treatment services, and developmental services.

Access to appropriate and quality health care is an important factor in the ability of the child welfare system to meet the needs of the abused and neglected children and youths it serves, whether the children and youths are in their own homes, in the homes of relatives, or in out-of-home care (i.e., family foster care, group care, or residential care).

Where there has been abuse or neglect, the child welfare system endeavors, whenever possible, to keep the family together and provide services to resolve the problems that led to the abuse or neglect. Supporting and stabilizing families so that they may remain together may hinge on adequate access to health care services for children and their parents. Too often, however, these services are nonexistent, inadequate to meet the demand, or inappropriate in light of the level of care or intensity of services that is needed, particularly in the area of mental health. Consequently, it may be difficult for child welfare agencies to effectively support families and stabilize situations to avoid family disruption.

As the number of reports of abuse and neglect continues to increase, so too does the number of children in out-of-home care. In 1990, some 407,000 children and youths were in out-of-home care. By the end of 1992, the number was approximately 442,000.[4] These children and youths likely have experienced significant abuse or neglect, tend to be extremely vulnerable, and often need a comprehensive range of health care services. Such youngsters often have histories of little or no health care and frequently suffer from a range of acute and chronic health conditions requiring medical attention. They are at high risk of mental health and developmental problems due to abuse and neglect, family instability, and, in many instances, exposure to alcohol or other drugs or HIV. Perhaps more than any other group of children, these youngsters require access to a comprehensive, coordinated array of physical health, mental health, and developmental services.

The present health care system, however, has proven inadequate in meeting the needs of this expanding population. Clearly, major changes are needed. As a starting point, the health care system, if it is to be truly responsive to vulnerable children and youths, must focus and be grounded on a recognition of certain basic principles:

- Children are dependent on others for their basic health care needs. Vulnerable children and youths who have experienced abuse or neglect are particularly dependent on caregivers to meet their primary and specialized health care needs, and, more than other children, must depend on individuals in their extended families and others to recognize their needs.

- It is the responsibility of parents, caregivers, and society as a whole to ensure that each child lives in an environment that daily promotes physical, intellectual, emotional, and social growth, and that assures each child the opportunity to develop into a physically and mentally healthy adult. Vulnerable children and youths who have experienced abuse and neglect are in particular need of a variety of opportunities for healthy growth and development.
- The growth and development of each child is multifaceted, involving physical, cognitive, and psychological components, all of which must be addressed as part of the health care system. Children and youths who have experienced abuse and neglect often have special needs, particularly in the areas of mental health and developmental services, because of prenatal, postnatal, familial, and social experiences. These needs must be addressed through a comprehensive, coordinated service delivery system.
- Children's individual physical, cognitive, and psychological needs must be met appropriately during each developmental stage. All children and youths should have access to health care services that foster their full potential through each developmental period. Vulnerable children and youths who have experienced abuse and neglect may require special health care services to ensure that developmental milestones are met.

The Status of Vulnerable Children

The children and youths served by the child welfare system are, for the most part, drawn from the ranks of children from low-income families, whose significantly compromised health status has been the focus of many reports. The results of these studies signal special concern for the health of the vulnerable children and youths in the child welfare system.

According to the U.S. Census Bureau, 13.8 million children—21 percent of all children under the age of 18—lived in poverty in 1992.[5,6] These children and youths are being debilitated by health conditions and problems that a responsive health care system could address and rectify. Recent statistics on children's health illustrate the dimensions of the problem:

- The infant mortality rate in 1990 was 9.2 deaths per 1,000 births. This rate had shown a rapid decline beginning in the 1960s but that decline slowed in the 1980s.[7]
- In 1990, 289,418 babies—7 percent of all live births—were born with low birthweight. The figure is the highest percentage of low birthweight babies since 1978.[8]
- Between 14 and 18 percent of all pregnancies involve prenatal exposure to alcohol or other drugs. Of that number, 4.5 percent involve cocaine exposure, 17.4 percent marijuana exposure, and 73 percent alcohol exposure.[9] According to recent estimates, 554,000 to 739,000 infants are exposed prenatally to illegal drugs each year.[10] Fetal alcohol syndrome affects one of every 600 to 750 children.[11]
- More than one-third of Caucasian children and over one-half of children of color ages one to four years have not been properly immunized against five common childhood diseases.[12]
- An estimated 12 million children, mostly poor, are at risk of lead poisoning. Exposure to lead stunts the intellectual growth of hundreds of thousands of youngsters each year.[13]
- The incidence of AIDS among infants, children, and adolescents continues to rise. As of March 1993, 5,647 cases of AIDS in persons younger than 20 years were reported to the Centers for Disease Control (CDC). The majority of pediatric AIDS cases result from prenatal transmission by mothers who are infected with HIV, with a disproportionate number of cases occurring among African American and Latino children. The statistics on pediatric AIDS cases, as reported to the CDC, do not include children and young people infected with HIV who are asymptomatic or in the early stages of the disease.[14]
- In 1990, 360,645 babies were born to single women under age 20, almost nine percent of all births that year. The percentage of all births to single teens increased 16 percent between 1985 and 1990.[15]
- Alcohol and other drugs continue to be widely used by young people. A study of high school seniors (class of 1990) found that 80.6 percent had used alcohol in the last year. An

additional 57.1 percent had used alcohol in the preceding month. The study also found that 33 percent of high school seniors surveyed reported using an illegal drug in the past year. Another 17 percent reported using an illegal drug at least once in the past month. Marijuana ranked as the most widely used illegal drug.[16]

These statistics detail a situation that is often exacerbated for children and youths in the child welfare system because of their heightened vulnerability to physical and mental health and developmental problems. For example:

- The fastest growing age group entering the child welfare system is children under two years, at least partly as a result of the drug epidemic that is leading to many infants who were prenatally exposed to alcohol and other drugs entering out-of-home care.[17]
- Children in out-of-home care are in poorer health than other children, and are more likely to suffer from a range of acute and chronic health problems.[18]
- Children entering out-of-home care now are more likely than those who entered care in 1984 to suffer from upper respiratory infections, dermatologic disorders, dental caries, and malnutrition.[19]
- Children and youths in the child welfare system suffer from a range of psychological and developmental problems leading to significant behavioral and emotional difficulties.[20]
- At least one-third of all substantiated cases of child abuse and neglect involve parental substance abuse, which is associated with higher risks of child abuse and neglect.[21]

Barriers to Health Care

As the above statistics reflect, the health status of vulnerable children demands a responsive health care program. The American health care system, however, clearly is not meeting the needs of these children and youths. Both financial and nonfinancial barriers to quality, comprehensive, and responsive health care limit the access of vulnerable children and youths to the services they need.

Financial Barriers

One of the most significant, if not the major, barrier to obtaining needed health care is financial: the lack of adequate health insurance. More and more families in the United States are finding themselves with no health insurance: families whose members are unemployed, families whose members are facing the prospect of unemployment, and families with employed members who cannot afford insurance or lack access to it. Data released by the U.S. Census Bureau reflect a continuing increase in the number of individuals without health insurance: in 1991, 35.2 million Americans had no insurance, as compared to 34.4 million in 1990.[22]

A significant number of children lack health insurance. In 1990, 12.9 percent of all children in the United States—almost nine million children—lacked health coverage at some point during the preceding year.[23] Parental employer-based health insurance, once a significant avenue for insuring against medical and health care costs, is no longer the resource that it once was for children. The proportion of children under the age of 18 that were covered by employer-based insurance at some point during the preceding year decreased from 72.8% to 61.5% between 1977 and 1991.[24] By 1987, almost 30% of all African American children and nearly 40% of Latino children in working, single parent families were totally uninsured at some point during the preceding year.[25] Children from low-income families are particularly affected. In 1991, 41 percent of such children under the age of 18 had no insurance.[26]

Even families who have some form of health insurance coverage may find that it does not cover many of the services they need. The mere presence of health insurance is not a guarantee of a reliable financial resource that will cover the costs of needed health care. Variations in insurance policies and practices, administrative complexity, and copayments create barriers to health care even when there is insurance coverage.

One response to the financial barriers to health care has been Medicaid, the federal-state financing system for health care designed to fill the gap for some low-income individuals who lack health insurance. Medicaid alone, however, is insufficient to resolve the problem. Although Medicaid provides health coverage for many low-income individuals, a significant number of Americans still lack access to adequate health care because they are ineligible for Medicaid. Even when individuals qualify for Medicaid benefits, they often find that the health care it makes available to them is inadequate. States vary substantially in the types of services they cover under their Medicaid programs and in the scope and duration of these services. The intrinsic limitations within the Medicaid system, based largely on its initial "welfare" link, further exacerbate the significant difficulties that many children and youths face in obtaining the health care they need.

Nonfinancial Barriers

Financial barriers related to the absence of insurance and to inadequate insurance coverage do not provide the sole explanation for the inadequate health care that vulnerable children, youths, and families often receive. Nonfinancial barriers to health care are equally problematic: inadequate transportation; language and cultural barriers that limit the ability of individuals to utilize existing resources; the maldistribution of physicians and other health care providers, particularly in inner cities and rural areas; and systems that fail to provide conveniently located facilities and flexible operating hours, or that lack the supportive services families need to effectively use health care services, such as child day care. Without attention to these factors, the provision of a financing mechanism for health care will fail to ensure access to needed health care.

The Response

The American health care delivery system must ensure that the physical, psychological, and developmental needs of all children and youths are met, particularly the needs of the vulnerable children, youths, and families served by the child welfare system. Currently, there are numerous proposals to reform the system. Some address specific needs of vulnerable children and youths, but none adequately responds to the wide range of needs of children and youths in the child welfare system. This document identifies the health care needs of the children and youths served by the child welfare system and the services that must be included in any benefit package for children and youths. It also identifies barriers to health care that must be addressed if the services contained in the benefit package are to be accessible to the most vulnerable in America.

Notes

1 National Committee for Prevention of Child Abuse, Center on Child Abuse Prevention Research, *Current Trends in Child Abuse Reporting and Fatalities: Results of the 1992 Annual Fifty State Study* (Chicago: National Committee for Prevention of Child Abuse, 1993).

[2] National Committee for Prevention of Child Abuse (1993).

[3] National Committee for Prevention of Child Abuse (1993).

[4] Voluntary Cooperation Information System (VCIS), *VCIS Research Notes* (Washington, DC: American Public Welfare Association, July 1993).

[5] United States Bureau of the Census, "Poverty in the United States: 1992," *Current Population Reports Series P60–185* (Washington, DC: U.S. Government Printing Office, 1993).

[6] U.S. Bureau of the Census (1993).

[7] National Center for Health Statistics, "Advance Report of Final Mortality Statistics, 1990," *Monthly Vital Statistics Report* 41, 7 (Supplement) (January 7, 1993).

[8] National Center for Health Statistics, "Advance Report of Final Natality Statistics, 1990," *Monthly Vital Statistics Report* 41, 9 (Supplement) (February 25, 1993).

[9] J.C. Burnison, Testimony Before the U.S. House of Representatives Select Committee on Narcotics Abuse and Control (July 30, 1991).

[10] D.S. Gromby and P. Shiono, "Estimating the Number of Substance Exposed Infants," *The Future of Children: Drug Exposed Infants* 1, 1 (Spring 1991): 17–25.

[11] A. Streissguth, "Fetal Alcohol Syndrome and the Teratogenicity of Alcohol: Policy Implications" (Prepared for the Eighth World Congress of the International Commission for the Prevention of Alcoholism and Drug Dependency, September, 1991), p. 7.

[12] Committee on Ways and Means, U.S. House of Representatives, Overview of Entitlement Reports (hereinafter "1993 Green Book") (Washington, DC: U.S. Government Printing Office, 1993), p. 1171.

[13] National Commission on Children, *Beyond Rhetoric: A New American Agenda for Children and Families* (Washington, DC: U.S. Government Printing Office, 1991), p. 121.

[14] U.S. Department of Health and Human Services, Centers for Disease Control. *HIV/AIDS Surveillance Reports* 5, 1 (May 1993).

[15] National Center for Health Statistics, "Advance Report of Final Natality Statistics, 1990."

16 L. Johnston, P. O'Malley, and J. Bachman, *Drug Use Among American High School Seniors, College Students and Young Adults, 1975–1990* (Rockville, MD: National Institute on Drug Abuse 1991).

17 L. Dunckel, ed., *Special Care: California's Children in Foster Care with Special Medical Needs* (Sacramento, CA: Children's Research Institute of California, 1989), pp. 1–27.

18 M.S. Wald, J.M. Carlsmith, and P.H. Liederman, *Protecting Abused/Neglected Children: A Comparison of Home and Foster Placement* (Palo Alto, CA: Stanford Center for the Study of Youth Development, 1985).

19 "Health Supervision of Children in Foster Care," Consensus Conference, New York State Department of Health and Social Services (June 6, 1990), p. 2.

20 D. Cicchetti and V. Carlson, *Child Maltreatment* (Cambridge, MA: Cambridge University Press, 1989), p. xv.

21 National Committee for Prevention of Child Abuse (1993).

22 1993 Green Book, p. 296.

24 *Child Protection Report* 18, 1 (Silver Spring, MD: Business Publishers, Inc., January 10, 1992), p. 4; *1993 Green Book*, p. 296.

25 *Child Protection Report* (1992), p. 5

26 *1993 Green Book*, p. 298.

The Benefit Package: Meeting the Needs of Vulnerable Children and Youths in the Child Welfare System

Introduction

The specific health service needs of the vulnerable children and youths served by the child welfare system can be divided into two major categories—primary and preventive health care, and specialized health care. Part One of this section examines the need for primary and preventive health care of three groups who are of particular concern to the child welfare community: (1) pregnant women; (2) infants, toddlers, and school-age children; and (3) adolescents. Part Two examines the specialized health care services that children and youths in the child welfare system need, specifically with regard to mental health, HIV infection and AIDS, and alcohol and other drug abuse.

Primary Health Care

Essentially, primary health care begins with services to pregnant women to provide the best opportunities for healthy fetal development and child well-being. Primary health care must include services for infants, toddlers, school-age children, and adolescents served by the child welfare system.

To maximize the health and well-being of newborns, an increasing number of whom are coming to the attention of the child welfare system, pregnant women must receive:

- Prenatal care, which must be available to all pregnant women regardless of income status.
- Nutrition services, which must be available to all pregnant women and to all children through age 12.
- Health education and counseling, including information regarding the effects of tobacco, alcohol, and other drug use during pregnancy, and the risks associated with HIV infection.

Infants, toddlers, and school-age children served by the child welfare system must receive:

- Primary health care services, including periodic examinations; vision, hearing, and dental screenings; health education; and immunizations.
- Early screening for disabling conditions, including lead poisoning and developmental delay.
- Mental health and developmental services, addressing the range of emotional and developmental conditions that children in the child welfare system experience.

Adolescents served by the child welfare system must receive:

- Primary health care services, including general health, vision, hearing, and dental screening; mental health screening; and health education.
- Reproductive health services specifically designed to address the issues of teenage pregnancy and sexually transmitted diseases.
- Mental health services, ranging from outpatient community-based services to residential care.

Specialized Health Care and Supportive Services

In addition to primary health care services, the children and youths served by the child welfare system must have access to specialized health care services, family-based services that support and enhance the health and well being of all family members, and services that address conditions associated with HIV and with alcohol and other drug exposure. Children and youths in the child welfare system must receive:

- Specialized health care services, including specialized medical treatment, rehabilitative services, and remedial care.
- Family support services to ensure and enhance the delivery and effectiveness of health care services.
- Services relating to HIV infection and AIDS, including voluntary testing for HIV, counseling, primary and specialized health care, case management, and coordination with community resources.
- Alcohol and other drug abuse prevention, support, and treatment services.
    - Alcohol or other drug abuse prevention and treatment services must be available and accessible to pregnant, postpartum, and parenting women, and should include preventive and educational services, outpatient services, residential treatment, and aftercare services.
    - A full array of physical health, mental health, and developmental services must be available and accessible to infants and children in the child welfare system who were exposed prenatally to alcohol or other drugs.
    - Chemically involved youths served by the child welfare system must have access to prevention and treatment services that include education, alcohol and other drug use prevention and counseling, treatment, rehabilitation and aftercare services.

PART I: PRIMARY HEALTH CARE

The World Health Organizations define *health* as "complete physical, mental and social well-being, not merely the absence of disease or infirmity."[1] Health promotion and disease prevention incorporate numerous factors, including health monitoring and professional services directed toward health maintenance.[2] Such services—usually referred to as primary health care—are particularly essential to the health of the vulnerable infants, toddlers, and school-age children served by the child welfare system.

Children and youths who have experienced abuse or neglect often have not had access to primary health care services. Financial barriers frequently pose significant obstacles to primary health care. Having few resources for primary and preventive health services and lacking health insurance, families may seek health care only in emergency situations.

Health insurance in and of itself, however, is no guarantee that vulnerable children and youths will have access to primary health care. A child may be eligible for Medicaid, for example, but the availability of primary care services may nevertheless be significantly limited. A state may not include a particular primary health service in its Medicaid plan, or there may be an inadequate number of providers to render services, a situation often associated with low reimbursement rates, particularly for obstetrical and pediatric services, and with the wide variance in Medicaid reimbursement rates for different types of health care services.

Primary health care service falls into two categories: primary and preventive care that must be available to meet the needs of all low-income children, youths, and pregnant women (the populations from which the children and youths served by the child welfare system primarily come), and primary health care that meets the specific needs of abused and neglected children and youths.

PRIMARY HEALTH CARE AND PREGNANT WOMEN

If the needs of young children who enter the child welfare system are to be met most effectively, it is first necessary to address the health care needs of their mothers during pregnancy. When pregnant women do not receive adequate prenatal care and nutrition, or when they engage in certain activities, their health status, as well as that of their children, is compromised. Their infants and children may suffer health and developmental problems on both a short- and long-term basis. Increasingly, the child welfare system is being asked to address the needs of these infants. The system is encountering a growing number of children with physical, mental, and developmental problems at or shortly after birth, problems that could be avoided or minimized with adequate, appropriate, and culturally sensitive prenatal care, nutrition services, and health care education and counseling for their mothers before and during pregnancy.

Prenatal Care

Prenatal care must be available to all pregnant women, regardless of income status.

The health consequences for infants as a result of insufficient prenatal care are well documented. Of particular relevance is the strong correlation between a mother's lack of adequate prenatal care and a baby's subsequent low birthweight, a condition associated with infant mortality and with poor health outcomes for the infant. A low birthweight infant (under 5.5 pounds) is 40 times more likely to die in the first month of life than a infant of average birthweight.[3] Low birthweight also correlates with health care complications and developmental problems, which in turn increase the infant's susceptibility to illness and developmental delay.

Infant mortality rates are particularly staggering among African American children, whose mothers are among those most likely to receive inadequate prenatal care or no prenatal care at all. As a result of inadequate prenatal care, African American children, as compared to Caucasian children, are twice as likely to be born weighing less than 2,500 grams and three times as likely to die during infancy.[4] Newborns of adolescent mothers who did not obtain prenatal care are also at particular risk.[5]

Appropriate and accessible prenatal care services can remedy this situation. Studies have shown that women who receive prenatal counseling, education, and health management have a significantly decreased risk of delivering infants of low birthweight.[6]

Nutrition

Nutrition services must be available to all pregnant women and to all children through the age of 12 years.

A woman's diet during pregnancy affects her child's development before and after birth. Without a sufficiently nutritious diet, pregnant women are more likely to give birth to low weight babies who, because of nutrition deficits during gestation, may experience a variety of health problems such as iron deficiency, growth retardation, and functional and cognitive disabilities. In addition, even children who were not affected by prenatal nutrition deficits may experience health and development problems if their own nutrition is inadequate. Proper nutrition is critical to infants and children because it directly affects developing brain functioning and physiologic growth.

The Supplemental Food Program for Women, Infants and Children (WIC) Program is one model for delivering nutrition services that support healthy development and functioning. This program could be used to expand nutrition services to all pregnant women and to children through age 12. Currently, the WIC program supplies food and nutrition education to low-income women who are pregnant or breast feeding and to children up to the age of five years who are considered at risk of poor nutrition. Studies have shown that a pregnant woman's participation in WIC decreases the risk that she will deliver prematurely or give birth to a low birthweight baby, and decreases the likelihood of fetal death.[7] The receipt of WIC benefits not only improves a mother's nutrition status but has been shown to increase the likelihood that she will seek prenatal care, will immunize her children, and will obtain regular pediatric care for her children.[8]

Health Education and Counseling

All pregnant women must have access to health education and counseling regarding the effects of tobacco, alcohol, and other drugs during pregnancy and the risks associated with HIV infection.

Cigarette smoking, consumption of alcoholic beverages, other drug use, and HIV infection during pregnancy jeopardize the current and long-term health of both the mother and her child. All foods, liquids, and drugs ingested by a pregnant woman can cross the placenta and enter the bloodstream of the developing fetus, exposing the infant to potential short- and long-term harm.[9] The child welfare system is serving a growing number of infants and young children whose physical and developmental status has been compromised by prenatal exposure to a variety of substances and conditions and who, as a result, are at heightened risk of abuse, neglect, and abandonment.

Smoking During Pregnancy. The use of tobacco by pregnant women has been directly linked to low birthweight and physical and developmental complications for their infants.[10] It is suspected that when nicotine crosses into the fetus' bloodstream, it causes blood vessels to constrict, reducing the amount of oxygen available and depleting the oxygen supply to the brain and the rest of the body. Approximately one-third of all pregnant women smoke cigarettes at the onset of pregnancy and 25 percent continue to smoke throughout their pregnancy.[11] Tobacco use occurs with greatest frequency among young and poor women. Infants born to women who smoke are at heightened risk of dying within the first year of life; those who survive may experience behavioral problems, slow cognitive development, and growth deficiency as they age.[12]

Alcohol and Other Drug Use During Pregnancy. Alcohol consumption during pregnancy directly affects the health of the developing fetus and is linked to miscarriage, low birthweight, growth retardation, and a shortened gestation period.[13] Fetal Alcohol Syndrome (FAS), a condition marked by prenatal and postnatal growth retardation, central nervous system disorders, and abnormal craniofacial features, affects as many as three out of every 1,000 infants and is the leading cause of preventable birth defects.[14] Many other children whose mothers used alcohol during pregnancy may suffer from Fetal Alcohol Effect (FAE), a condition that is not as pronounced as FAS but that has serious consequences for the child's physical, emotional, and intellectual development.[15]

Use of drugs other than alcohol during pregnancy also poses a serious—and sometimes lethal—threat to the health of the developing fetus. Drug use by pregnant women is linked to serious nutrition problems, poor pregnancy outcomes, health crises leading to emergency room visits, and addictive behaviors that impair judgment and heighten the risk that the woman will engage in high-risk sexual activity.[16] Like alcohol and nicotine, cocaine and other drugs can cross the placenta and enter the fetal circulatory system. Fetal drug exposure results in fetal blood vessel constriction, leading to insufficient oxygen flow, a decrease in nutrients, brain damage and developmental delay, abnormalities of fetal organs and extremities, and possible infant addiction. Children who are exposed prenatally to drugs may be physically and developmentally fragile, and will likely be in need of expensive intensive care and attention as newborns.

Alcohol and other drug-affected infants are at heightened risk of abuse and neglect. In a study by the Child Welfare League of America, 254 public and private child welfare agencies responded to questions relating to the impact of alcohol and other drugs on children and their families, and on rates of child abuse and neglect. Public sector child welfare agencies reported that 37 percent of the children they served during fiscal year 1990 were affected by problems associated with alcohol or other drugs; private sector child welfare agencies reported that 57.4 percent of the children they served were affected by alcohol or other drugs. Overall, 93 percent of the agencies reported that they were seeing more children and youths for whom problems related to alcohol and other drugs were factors in the initial investigation of child abuse and neglect.[17]

HIV Infection and AIDS. The incidence of HIV infection and AIDS continues to rise in the United States, with children experiencing the greatest increase. Pregnant women, in particular, need special counseling because of the possibility of their own HIV infection and the likelihood that HIV will be perinatally transmitted to their infants.[18] HIV infection among women is often associated with drug use, and counseling must address both factors. Studies reflect that 72 percent of women who are HIV infected are intravenous drug users themselves or the sexual partners of intravenous drug users, and 51 percent of children born with HIV infection were born to mothers who were themselves drug involved.[19] It is essential that women who engage in intravenous drug abuse or sexual relations with an IV drug user receive counseling regarding the dangers involved with the use of drugs and unprotected sexual intercourse, including the potential impact on their children.

PRIMARY HEALTH CARE AND INFANTS, TODDLERS, AND SCHOOL-AGED CHILDREN

The child welfare system serves some of the most vulnerable infants, toddlers, and children in America. These children have experienced abuse, neglect, and abandonment and are at particular risk of physical health, mental health, and developmental problems. The child welfare system serves infants, toddlers, and children in a variety of settings: in their own homes, in out-of-home care settings such as family foster homes, and in settings in which they are awaiting adoptive placements or have been placed with adoptive families. In each instance, children who have been abused or neglected need a wide range of health care services. Some of these services are needed because of the special vulnerabilities of these children; others parallel the services needed by all children.

Primary Health Care

Primary health care services, including physical examinations; screening for vision, hearing, and dental status; health education; and immunizations must be available to all children served by the child welfare system.

Although the American Academy of Pediatrics recommends that children from birth to six years of age visit a pediatrician periodically, even when healthy, so that they receive health monitoring and health maintenance services,[20] many children do not receive such services. A 1986 study found that 37 percent of families with incomes below the poverty line reported that their children between the ages of one and five years had not visited a physician within the previous year.[21] Studies consistently reflect that children living above the poverty level are significantly more likely to have seen a doctor than those living below that level.[22] Continuous care from a single provider is less available for children from low-income families and, as a result, they are less likely to be seen by a provider who knows their individual needs, circumstances, and health history, and more likely to be seen in hospital emergency rooms.[23]

To some degree, this lack of access correlates with health insurance. In one study, for example, 53 percent of uninsured children had not seen a pediatrician within the previous year, compared to only 16 percent of the children covered by private insurance.[24]

Children served by the child welfare system tend to be less healthy than other children and more likely to experience acute and chronic health problems and disabling conditions.[25] These may be avoided or the consequences limited through the provision of early and comprehensive primary health care services.

A variety of physical health care services to protect and promote physical well-being and enhance the quality of life for vulnerable infants, toddlers, and school age children must be available.

Health Examinations Screening for Vision, Hearing and Dental Status. Children served by the child welfare system need regular and periodic physical examinations to preserve health, prevent illness, identify problems as early as possible, and correct conditions that can cause physical, cognitive, and psychological problems later in life. Likewise, early and periodic screening for vision, hearing, and dental status are essential to detecting problems early and providing early intervention.

Health Education. Health education is an equally essential health service for vulnerable children. Health education must include the promotion of sound nutrition and exercise to avoid future problems such as obesity, anemia, high blood pressure, and heart disease. It must also incorporate efforts to prevent childhood accidents and injuries, including car accidents, drowning, bicycle accidents, fire, and accidental poison and drug ingestion, the most common sources of preventable injury to infants, toddlers, and children.[26] Education for caregivers, including biological parents, foster parents, and adoptive parents, is equally important for the promotion of children's health and recognition of risks to normal development and growth.

Immunizations. A critical component of primary health care is the timely administration of immunizations. Vaccinations can prevent eight communicable childhood diseases: diphtheria, tetanus, measles, polio, rubella, mumps, congenital rubella, and pertussis. Preschool-age children are among those most vulnerable to these diseases, and are disproportionately affected by these conditions. Large numbers of children, however, including those served by the child welfare system, do not receive the necessary vaccination series. For example, over the past three years, measles—a preventable disease—has affected more than 55,000 individuals and in 1990, caused the deaths of 89 persons.[27]

Early Screening for Disabling Conditions

Screening for lead poisoning and developmental delay are essential services for all children served by the child welfare system.

A growing number of infants, toddlers, and school-age children have been exposed to environmental hazards such as lead, or were exposed prenatally to alcohol and other drugs, heightening the need for screening services for congenital problems, developmental delay, and physical and mental disabilities.

Screening for Lead Poisoning. Children served by the child welfare system may be particularly at risk of lead poisoning because they have lived in substandard housing and because they are at heightened risk of inadequate nutrition, a condition that often contributes to lead poisoning. Approximately 12 million children, most living in inner cities, are exposed to dangerous levels of lead and are at risk of serious health problems, including physical and developmental problems.[28] Because lead poisoning results from long-term, low-level exposure that cumulatively results in clinical toxicity, routine and periodic testing of children's blood is essential to detect exposure, provide the necessary management, and prevent further exposure.

Screening for Developmental Conditions. Infants, toddlers, and school-age children served by the child welfare system are at risk of physical and mental disabilities that can have a serious long-term effect on their lives. These conditions are often associated with poor nutrition, environmental and emotional deprivation, alcohol and other drug exposure, HIV infection, and other conditions that develop during gestation and early infancy, or that are the result of family stress or disruption. Early and periodic screening for developmental delays and physical and mental conditions is particularly essential for this group of children, and must be systematically implemented and promoted through outreach activities, particularly for children who are geographically and/or socially isolated.

Mental Health and Developmental Services

A full array of mental health and developmental services must be available to the infants, toddlers, and children served by the child welfare system.

Between 12 and 15 percent of all American children—some 7.5 to 9.5 million youngsters—suffer from some form of mental disorder.[29] Although it is not known how many of these children are being served by the child welfare system, studies have demonstrated that children who have been abused and neglected and who are placed in out-of-home care have high rates of emotional, behavioral, and developmental problems,[30] and that maltreatment of children closely correlates with mental health problems.[31] Studies have found that when children in out-of-home care are assessed for psychological problems, between 35 percent and 95 percent are found to be moderately to severely impaired.[32] Problems often include adjustment reactions, academic problems, self-destructiveness and aggression, poor self-esteem, depression, and impaired interpersonal relationships.[33] Developmental problems are also common.[34] As understanding of the mental health problems of children in out-of-home care has improved, child welfare practitioners have recognized that, although children in the child welfare system require a wide range of mental health services,[35] they often do not receive them.[36] The short- and long-term effects of abuse, neglect, and abandonment on infants, toddlers, and school-age children require that those services be available and accessible to ensure early and effective intervention.

Primary Health Care and Adolescents

Adolescence as a developmental phase is marked by physical, intellectual, and emotional changes that require a range of health care services.

As compared to other age groups, adolescents are more likely to be sexually, physically, and emotionally abused.[42] Adolescents who enter the child welfare system are particularly vulnerable to health problems because they have experienced not only the turbulence associated with the developmental tasks of adolescence, but also have been exposed to abuse, neglect, or exploitation that can seriously undermine their well-being. These young people need primary health care services, reproductive health services, and mental health assessments and services.

Primary Health Care Services

Primary health care services, including general health, vision, hearing, and dental screenings; mental health screening; and health education, must be available and accessible to all adolescents served by the child welfare system.

Like younger children, adolescents have an ongoing need for primary health care services, including general health, vision, hearing, and dental screenings; mental health screening; and health education. These services, especially health education, are essential to improving the health status of adolescents and preventing problems and conditions that could significantly impact their well-being, such as accidental injuries, cancer, heart disease, obesity, anemia, fatigue, chemical dependency, and HIV infection.[43] Likewise, periodic mental health assessments are critical to the well-being of adolescents. Such assessments allow early identification of depression or mental illness that can lead to suicidal, destructive, or violent behavior. Adolescents in the child welfare system are particularly susceptible to physical and mental health problems, as they have likely experienced abuse and neglect, lived on the street as runaways or homeless youths, and suffered physical and sexual exploitation.

Adolescents often lack primary and preventive health care, frequently as a result of having no health insurance. In 1990, 14 percent of all teens had no primary source of health care, while 30 percent of adolescents aged 12 to 17 reported that they had not seen a physician over the previous year.[44] Adolescents are less likely to utilize private, office-based primary care physicians than any other age group, averaging only 1.6 visits per person per year.[45] Teens whose families have incomes below the poverty line more frequently report fair or poor health than do those from families with incomes above the poverty line.[46] Children and adolescents from families earning less than $35,000, as compared to teens in families with higher incomes, for example, have 1.7 times more short-term hospital stays and miss 1.4 times more days from school because of illness.[47]

Reproductive Health Services

Health care services specifically designed to address issues of sexuality, teenage pregnancy, and sexually transmitted diseases must be available and accessible to all adolescents served by the child welfare system.

Adolescents served by the child welfare system are particularly in need of reproductive health services because they frequently have histories of physical and sexual abuse and exploitation. These services must be designed and delivered in ways that recognize the specific needs, concerns, and attitudes of young people.

Teenage Pregnancy. Since 1973, approximately one million teenage pregnancies have occurred each year.[48] Over 27,000 of the total number of teenage pregnancies were to women under age 15.[49] Women who give birth before age 18 are at increased risk of health and birth complications, and have a reduced probability of finishing high school.[50] Teenage pregnancy and motherhood often place young women in a role for which they are emotionally, psychologically, socially, and educationally unprepared. Premature parenthood interrupts the adolescent's normal development and transition into young adulthood. Equally troubling is the finding that the infants of adolescent mothers are at greater risk for illness and birth defects.[51] Studies show that the infants born to unmarried teenagers are 1.5 times more likely to die in infancy and twice as likely to be born underweight than those born to women age 20 or older.[52]

Unintended pregnancy and parenthood among teenagers places them under financial and emotional stress and heightens the risk that their children will be abandoned, abused, or neglected.[53] Stress on adolescent mothers may increase when HIV infection affects the mother and/or infant, or the infant is exposed prenatally to alcohol or other drugs and requires specialized health care. The interaction of adolescent sexuality activity and pregnancy, alcohol and drug use, and HIV infection, on the one hand, and the increased risks of child abuse and neglect, on the other hand, have serious implications for the child welfare system.

Child welfare agencies must be able to respond in a variety of ways. In some cases, both the adolescent mother and her infant may need out-of-home care, including primary and specialized health care services. In other situations, the child welfare system may serve the young mother and her child in their own home, mobilizing the needed resources to keep the young family intact. In yet other cases, the infant and adolescent mother may need to be separated in order to meet the infant's special needs and assist the mother in obtaining the help she needs.

In addition, studies suggest that young people in out-of-home care may be particularly susceptible to sexual activity and its consequences of unintended pregnancy. A Westat study of young people who had exited care found that 42 percent of youths surveyed had either given birth to or fathered a child.[54] Sixty percent of the females in out-of-home care had given birth, however, but only 24 percent of the males had fathered a child, suggesting that gender is a key factor in developing programs that assist youths in avoiding early parenthood.[55]

The vulnerability of women who have been in out-of-home care persists after they leave care. A Westat follow-up study found that over 60 percent of the young women had at least one child two to four years after discharge from out-of-home care, while by contrast, only 25 percent of the general population aged 18 to 24 had given birth.[56] Another study of young women aged 13 to 18 found that those in out-of-home care, including family foster care, were 50 percent more likely to report having sex and were significantly less informed about birth control than those not in care.[57]

These findings emphasize the need for preventive reproductive health services for youths served by the child welfare system. Studies of the effectiveness of family planning services have demonstrated that counseling, education, and increased access to contraception for sexually active adolescents can have a positive effect on deterring unwanted teenage pregnancy and improving the health of the mother and her child. One study of teenage women involved with family planning programs, for example, found that unintended pregnancy rates, births, abortions, and miscarriages decreased when such services were made available.[58] Preventive services that address factors associated with teenage pregnancy—limited education, lower socioeconomic status, inadequate nutrition, smoking, and abuse of alcohol and other drugs—have been found to be effective in reducing the rate of teenage pregnancy.[59]

Sexually Transmitted Diseases. Adolescents often engage in sexual activities that place them at risk for sexually transmitted diseases (STDs). Sexual activity among adolescents is often associated with alcohol or other drug use; psychological factors such as low self-esteem, anxiety, feelings of powerlessness or rebelliousness; peer acceptance; and failure to fully appreciate the consequences of behavior.[60] Age 13 is a particularly critical age, often marking the onset of sexual behavior.[61]

The need for reproductive health services targeted to STDs is well documented by statistical rates of teenage sexual activity and STDs. Approximately one-fourth of 15-year-old girls and one-third of 15-year-old boys have become sexually active.[62] More than half of all sexually active teens fail to use contraception when they first engage in intercourse,[63] placing them at heightened risk of pregnancy and sexually transmitted diseases, including HIV. Approximately 2.5 million adolescents report having contracted a STD, with approximately 25 percent reporting that they contracted the STD prior to high school graduation.[64] Studies reflect that rates of STDs are rising among adolescents. The incidence of gonorrhea among sexually active teens ages 15 to 19, for example, surpasses that of young adults ages 20 to 24.[65]

Mental Health Services

An array of mental health services for adolescents, ranging from outpatient community-based services to residential treatment, must be available and accessible to the youths served by the child welfare system.

Because of the powerful physiological, psychological, and interpersonal changes that mark adolescence, teenagers in particular are at risk of some type of mental health problem, ranging from mild adjustment reactions to more serious emotional and behavioral difficulties. Changes in peer groups and family structure, the academic and social dynamics of high school, identity questioning and introspection, and possible experimentation with alcohol, drugs, and sex may contribute to the confusion, anxiety, and stress adolescents experience. Withdrawal from families, friends, and teachers, and feelings of isolation and loneliness may occur, leading to depression and, in some cases, suicidal thinking.

The stress associated with the usual developmental milestones during adolescence may be heightened for youths in the child welfare system because of experiences related to abuse or neglect, sexual exploitation, running away, alcohol or other drug involvement, sexual orientation concerns, and social and academic difficulties. These youngsters often include the approximately 1.2 million children who run away each year and the teens seen at shelters, where three-quarters report being victims of physical or sexual abuse.[66] These teens are particularly susceptible to suicidal thinking and behavior, the second leading cause of death (after accidents) among teens.[67] In addition to the almost 5,000 teens who take their lives through suicide each year, there is evidence that eight times as many teens unsuccessfully attempt suicide.[68] Between 12 and 15 percent of all adolescents suffer from significant mental disorders; the percentage is believed to be higher for adolescents served by the child welfare system. As many as 70 percent of children and youths who need mental services, however, do not receive them.[69]

Early mental health assessment and intervention are essential for adolescents, particularly those served by the child welfare system. They must include counseling for alcohol and drug abuse, depression, sexual or physical abuse, sexual orientation issues, and family problems. Mental health services of varying degrees of intensity must be available. For most adolescents who need mental health services, short-term counseling and support is the appropriate service response. For some teens, however, more intensive intervention is required in the form of day treatment, partial hospitalization, or short-term and long-term residential treatment. Services must incorporate peer counseling, group support, and individualized therapeutic services specifically designed to meet the mental health needs of adolescents in a way that adolescents can accept and use them.

Notes

1 L. Breslow, "A Health Promotion Primer for the 1990s," *Health Affairs* 9, 2 (Summer 1990): 9.

2 Breslow (1990): 19.

3 National Institute of Medicine, *Preventing Low Birthweight* (Washington, DC: National Academy Press 1985), pp. 27–29.

4 National Commission on Children, *Beyond Rhetoric: A New American Agenda for Children and Families* (Washington, DC: U.S. Government Printing Office, 1991), p. 162.

5 F. Hechniger, *Fateful Choices, Healthy Youth for the 21st Century* (New York: Carnegie Corporation of New York, 1992), p. 77.

6 U.S. Congress, Office of Technology Assessment, *Healthy Children: Investing in the Future* (Washington, DC: U.S. Government Printing Office, 1988).

7 D. Rush, *National Evaluation of the Special Supplemental Food Program for Women, Infants and Children*, vol. 1 (Washington, DC: U.S. Government Printing Office, 1986).

8 Rush (1986).

9 B. Zuckerman, "Drug-Exposed Infants: Understanding the Medical Risk," *The Future of Children: Drug-Exposed Infants* 1, 1 (Spring 1991): 27.

10 J.C. Kleinman and A. Kopstein, "Smoking During Pregnancy, 1967-1980." *American Journal of Public Health* 77 (1987): 823–25

11 *Vital and Health Statistics*, series 10, no. 163 (Hyattsville, MD: Department of Health and Human Services, DHHS Pub. No. (PHS) 88-1591, 1988).

12 J.C. Kleinman and J.H. Madans, "The Effects of Maternal Smoking, Physical Stature and Educational Attainment on the Incidence of Low Birthweight." *American Journal of Epidemiology* 6, 121 (1985): 832–55.

13 H.L. Rosett and L. Weiner, *Alcohol and the Fetus: A Clinical Perspective* (New York: Oxford University Press, 1984), p. 19.

14 A. Streissguth and S. Ramdels, "Long-Term Effects of Fetal Alcohol Syndrome" in *Alcohol and Child/Family Health*, edited by G.C. Robinson and R.W. Armstrong (Vancouver, BC: University of British Columbia, 1988), p. 135.

15 A. Streissguth, "Fetal Alcohol Syndrome and the Teratogenicity of Alcohol: Policy Implications" (Prepared for the Eighth World Congress of the International Commission for the Prevention of Alcoholism and Drug Dependency, September 1991), p. 7.

16 L.G. Keith, S.N. McGregor, and J.J. Sciara, "Drug Use in Pregnancy," in *Drugs, Alcohol, Pregnancy and Parenting*, edited by I.J. Chasnoff (Hingham, MA: Kluwer Academic Publishers, 1988).

17 North American Commission on Chemical Dependency and Child Welfare, *Children at the Front: A Different View of the War on Alcohol and Drugs* (Washington, DC: Child Welfare League of America 1992), pp. 176–177.

18 D. Albritten, *Children with HIV/AIDS: A Sourcebook for Caring* (Alexandria, VA: National Association of Children's Hospitals and Related Institutions, 1990), p. 203.

19 Albritten (1990).

20 National Center for Children in Poverty, *Alive and Well? A Research and Policy Review of Health Programs for Poor Young Children* (New York: Columbia University, 1991), p. 85.

21 National Center for Children in Poverty, *Alive and Well?* (1991).

22 National Center for Children in Poverty, *Five Million Children, A Statistical Profile of Our Poorest Young Citizens* (New York: Columbia University, 1990), p. 63.

23 National Center for Children in Poverty, *Five Million Children* (1990), p. 63.

24 National Center for Children in Poverty, *Five Million Children* (1990), p. 69.

25 H. Dubowitz, *The Physical and Mental Health and Educational Status of Children Placed with Relatives—Final Report.* (Baltimore, MD: School of Medicine, University of Maryland at Baltimore, 1990).

26 U.S. Department of Health and Human Services, Public Health Service, *Healthy People 2000: National Health Promotion and Disease PRevention Objectives* (Washington, DC: U.S. Government Printing Office, 1991)

27 J. Liu and S. Rosenbaum, *Medicaid and Childhood Immunizations: A National Study* (Washington, DC: Children's Defense Fund, 1992), p. i.

28 Centers for Disease Control, "Fatal Pediatric Poisoning from Leaded Paint—Wisconsin 1990," *Morbidity and Mortality Weekly Report* 40 (March 29, 1991): 193–195.

29 U.S. Congress, Office of Technology Assessment, *Children's Mental Health: Problems and Services—Background Paper* (Washington, DC: U.S. Government Printing Office, 1986), pp. 4–5; *Final Report: Community-Based Mental Health Services for Children in the Child Welfare System*, vol. 1 (Calverton, MD: Macro, International Inc., Contract No. HHS-100-91-0016-01, June 30, 1992), p. v.

30 N.J. Hochstadt, P.K. Jaudes, and K.A. Zimo, "The Medical and Psychological Needs of Children Entering Foster Care," *Child Abuse and Neglect* 11 (1987):

53–62; A. McIntyre and T.Y. Keesler, "Psychological Disorders among Foster Children," *Clinical Journal of Child Psychology* 15, 4 (1986): 297–303.

[31] D. Fanshel, S.J. Finch, and J.F Grundy, "Foster Children in the Life-Course Perspective: The Casey Program Experience," *Child Welfare* LXVIII, 5 (September–October 1989): 467–478.

[32] E.L. Schor, "Foster Care," *Pediatrics Review* 10 (1989): 209–216; M. Swire and F. Kaveler, "The Health Status of Foster Children," *Child Welfare* LVI, 10 (December 1977): 635–655.

[33] Dubowitz (1990).

[34] M.D. Simms, "The Foster Care Clinic: A Community Program to Identify Treatment Needs of Children in Foster Care," *Journal of Development and Behavioral Pediatrics* 10, 3 (1989): 121–128.

[35] N. Halfon, G. Berkowitz, and L. Klee, "Mental Health Service Utilization by Children in Foster Care in California," *Pediatrics* 89, 6 (June 1992): 1238; E.L. Schor, "Foster Care," *Peds Clin NA* 35 (1988): 1241–52.

[36] Dubowitz (1990); Hochstadt et al. (1987); Simms (1989).

[37] Shor (1988); Halfon (1992).

[38] National Commission on Child Welfare and Family Preservation, *A Commitment to Change* (Washington, DC: American Public Welfare Association, 1991), p. 4.

[39] Voluntary Cooperative Information System VCIS, *VCIS Research Notes* (Washington, DC: American Public Welfare Association, 1993).

[40] Hochstadt et al. (1987); Dubowitz (1990).

[41] Child Welfare League of America, *Standards for Health Care Services for Children in Out-of-Home Care* (Washington, DC: Child Welfare League of America, 1988), pp. 19–38.

[42] National Center on Child Abuse and Neglect. *Study of National Incidence of Child Abuse and Neglect: 1988* (Washington, DC: U.S. Department of Health and Human Services).

[43] Hechniger (1992), pp. 21–45.

[44] Hechniger (1992), pp. 38–39, citing National Commission on the Role of the School and the Community in Improving Adolescent Health, *Code Blue: Uniting for a Healthier Youth* (Alexandria VA: National Association of State Boards of Education, and Chicago, IL: American Medical Association, 1990).

[45] "Health Care Reform: How Do Women, Children and Teens Fare?" Hearing before the Select Committee on Children, Youth and Families, United States House of Representatives, 102nd Congress, 2d Sess. May 5, 1992 (Washington, DC: U.S. Government Printing Office, 1992), p. 6.

[46] Hechniger (1992), pp. 38–39, citing *Code Blue.*

[47] Hechniger (1992), pp. 38–39, citing *Code Blue.*

[48] Committee on Ways and Means, U.S. House of Representatives, Overview of Entitlement Reports (hereinafter "1993 Green Book") (Washington, DC: U.S. Government Printing Office, 1993), p. 1138.

[49] 1993 Green Book, p. 1138.

[50] Hechniger (1992), pp. 76-78.

[51] Hechniger (1992), p. 77.

[52] National Commission on Children (1991), p. 162.

[53] Hechniger (1992), p. 76.

[54] Westat, Inc., *A National Evaluation of Title IV-E Foster Care Independent Living Programs for Youth, Final Report,* Phase 2, vol. 1 (Rockville, MD: Westat, Inc., 1991), pp. 3–20.

[55] Westat (1991).

[56] Westat (1991), p. xv.

[57] *A Decade of Denial: Teens and AIDS in America,* A Report of the Select Committee on Children, Youth and Families, United States House of Representatives, 102nd Congress, 2d Session (Washington, DC: U.S. Government Printing Office, 1992), p. xviii.

[58] Hechniger (1992), pp. 101–106.

[59] Hechniger (1992), pp. 70–106.

[60] Hechniger (1992), pp. 79–80.

[61] C. Carpenter, B. Glassner, B. Johnson, and J. Loughlin, *Kids, Drugs and Crime* (Lexington, MA: Lexington Books, 1988), p. 120.

[62] Hechniger (1992), p. 72.

[63] Hechniger (1992), p. 73.

[64] Hechniger (1992), p. 74.

[65] Hechniger (1992), p. 74.

[66] A. Rosewater, "Child and Family Trends: Beyond the Numbers," in *Caring for America's Children,* edited by F. Maccchiarola (Proceedings of the Academy of Political Science, 1989), p. 15.

[67] M.L. Rosenberg, J.C. Smith, L.E. Davidson, and J.M. Conn, "The Emergence of Youth Suicide: An Epidemiological Analysis and Public Health Perspective," *Annual Review of Public Health* 8 (1987): 417–440.

[68] Rosenberg et al. (1987).

[69] U.S. Congress, Office of Technology Assessment, *Children's Mental Health.*

Part 2: Specialized Health Care and Supportive Services

In addition to primary health care services, children and youths served by the child welfare system often need specialized health care services. These children and youths, whether they are served in their own homes, in out-of-home care, or in adoptive placements, may have special health care needs related to medically complex or disabling conditions, exposure to HIV, or chemical involvement. The health care system must provide specialized services that appropriately address all of these needs.

Specialized Health Care

Specialized medical treatment, rehabilitative services, and remedial care must be available and accessible to the children and youths served by the child welfare system.

In 1988, nearly 20 million children under the age of 18 had one or more chronic illnesses requiring specialized medical care and rehabilitative and remedial services.[1] Although children not in care also experience such problems, those in the child welfare system are more likely to have serious illnesses and higher rates of certain conditions and disabilities. Infant and child mortality, Sudden Infant Death Syndrome (SIDS), and unintended injuries occur at higher rates among poor children than among non-poor children,[2] and as a result, tend to occur at significant rates among children and youths in the child welfare system.

The emotional and financial strains associated with a child's condition may create stresses that place a family at risk of disruption. The health care system, as an important element in efforts to support and strengthen families, must offer an array of affordable and accessible specialized services to meet the more complex health care needs of the children and youths it serves. These services must include specialized medical treatment, rehabilitative services, and remedial care. Too often, however, health care services for specialized conditions are absent, inaccessible, or too costly.

Likewise, children and youths placed in out-of-home care frequently suffer from health conditions that require specialized medical attention and rehabilitative services. Because they often have experienced significant abuse and neglect, these youngsters tend to be among the most vulnerable and fragile children and youths. Youngsters with disabilities who are cared for in out-of-home settings, such as family foster care and group residential care, often require specialized services to ensure maximum physical and mental growth and development. An array of rehabilitative, remedial, and supportive services—including physical therapy, speech therapy, occupational therapy and assistive technology—is often needed to remedy or minimize the effects of illness and disability.

SERVICES RELATING TO HIV AND AIDS

An array of services related to Human Immunodeficiency Virus (HIV) and Acquired Immune Deficiency Syndrome (AIDS) must be available to the children, youths, and families served by the child welfare system, including voluntary testing for HIV, counseling, primary and specialized health care, case management, and coordination with community resources.

Services related to HIV and AIDS are of growing importance to women and children, who are being affected in increasing numbers by the disease.

Pregnant Women and Newborn Infants

The number of HIV-positive pregnant women continues to grow. As a result, so too does the number of HIV-positive infants and children. Approximately 1,800 to 3,000 infants who are later determined to be HIV infected are born annually, and the Centers for Disease Control (CDC) estimated that over 20,000 children had been infected with HIV by the end of 1991.[3] Most of the infants who prove to be HIV infected contract the virus from their mothers, primarily through in utero transmission. Maternal HIV infection and drug use are closely related: the majority of pregnant women who are HIV infected use drugs intravenously or have sexual contact with an intravenous drug user.[4] Because of the connection between HIV infection and drug use, newborns may be dually exposed to HIV and drugs and experience significant health problems at birth.[5]

When mothers of newborns are debilitated by both HIV and drug use, their children may be at particular risk. The newborn's physical and emotional needs may be more than the mother can meet, particularly when the child is medically fragile. Child welfare professionals are finding that children who test positive for HIV, and children whose mothers are HIV infected, are at greater risk of abandonment, neglect, physical abuse, and serious illness than are those children for whom HIV has not affected mother or child.

Infants and Children

The effect of HIV upon an infant's or child's immune system is devastating, and can lead to multiple health complications, including failure to thrive, cancer, loss of sight, neurological impairment, and developmental disabilities.[6] Children who are HIV infected who survive early infancy must be monitored carefully for the appearance of HIV symptoms and/or the onset of AIDS, so that appropriate medical interventions may be initiated as quickly as possible to control, to the maximum extent, the effects of the disease.[7]

HIV infection and AIDS place significant financial, emotional, and physical demands upon parents and caregivers. Because of the frailty of their condition, infants and children who are HIV infected require special attention, primary and specialized medical care, frequent physician visits, special medication in some cases, and in all instances, supportive services for both the child and family, including respite care, counseling, and referral and linkage with community resources. The challenges of caring for a child who is also HIV infected are significant for any caregiver, but may be overwhelming to a parent who is HIV infected, is drug involved, or lacks financial and social supports. Because of the family circumstances often associated with HIV, infants and children who are HIV infected are at risk of abandonment, abuse, and neglect, and thus may enter the child welfare system.

Of growing concern to the child welfare community are the infants with HIV infection who are entering the out-of-home care system, including a new population of *border babies*—infants in hospitals who are medically cleared for discharge but cannot leave because their parent(s) cannot be located or cannot assume responsibility for their care. These infants, like other children who are HIV infected, need caregivers who understand and are able to meet their needs, health care providers with expertise in pediatric HIV infection and AIDS, and the support of trained counselors with skills in locating and assisting parents who are drug dependent and/or HIV infected.

Adolescents

Teenagers and young adults, once not considered at significant risk for HIV infection, now squarely face the possibility of HIV infection and AIDS. Rates of HIV infection and AIDS are rising among adolescents and young adults who were infected during adolescence. As of March 1993, 1,167 cases of AIDS had been reported among teenagers and 10, 949 cases had been reported in young adults between the ages of 20 and 24.[8] Of all AIDS cases reported as of March 1993, one in five was among young adults in their twenties. Because of the average eight- to ten-year latency period for the disease, most of these persons were likely infected as teenagers. The impact of AIDS is perhaps most strikingly illustrated by the almost 70 percent increase in the total number of AIDS cases among young persons ages 13 to 24 years between April 1991 and March 1993.[9]

Despite uncertainty about the exact incidence of HIV infection among adolescents, recent research shows that at least two out of every 1,000 college students are infected with HIV.[10] Because AIDS has a latency period which may extend to ten years, there may be many other teens currently infected with HIV who remain unaware that they carry the virus and who may be infecting others.[11] Although 13 percent of the cases of AIDS among adolescents are attributed to personal intravenous drug use, 68 percent of adolescents with AIDS contracted the disease through sexual contact.[12] The teens at greatest risk of becoming infected with HIV are those whom the child welfare system is most likely to serve: runaways; intravenous drug users; those who have had multiple sexual partners and/or engage in unprotected sex, who have had homosexual experiences, or who have been involved in prostitution; and incarcerated teens.[13]

Alcohol and Other Drug Abuse Prevention and Treatment

Specialized services designed to prevent and treat alcohol and other drug abuse must be available and accessible to pregnant and parenting women who are chemically dependent, infants and children who are exposed to alcohol and other drugs, and chemically involved youths.

Pregnant and Parenting Women Who Abuse Alcohol or Other Drugs

A full array of alcohol or other drug abuse prevention and treatment services must be available and accessible to pregnant and postpartum women, including preventive and educational services, outpatient treatment services, residential treatment, and aftercare services.

The use of alcohol and other drugs by pregnant women poses a health threat to the mother and exposes the fetus to harmful substances that can have detrimental effects on the child's development. Each year, some 40,000 babies are born at risk of Fetal Alcohol Syndrome (FAS) or Fetal Alcohol Effects (FAE) because of their mothers' alcohol use during pregnancy.[14] Approximately five million women of childbearing age in the United States use illegal drugs.[15] Studies suggest between 14 and 18 percent of all pregnancies involve fetal alcohol or other drug exposure.[16]

Although the physiological effects of alcohol and other drug abuse may be limited to the mother and child, chemical dependency affects the entire family. Alcohol and drug use can impair a parent's ability to care for his or her child and may lead to abuse or neglect. Women who abuse alcohol or other drugs may already be vulnerable to stress. Studies suggest that as a group, chemically dependent women are likely to have experienced childhood sexual abuse, to be illiterate and/or unemployed, to have suffered from familial instability and violence, to have inadequate housing or face homelessness, and to suffer from a range of problems related to poverty and inadequate health care.[17] These problems may combine to create pressures that exacerbate existing emotional and psychological difficulties and affect the mother's ability to function as a parent. Findings that chemically dependent mothers tend to be less sensitive and responsive to their infants and to have less physical contact with them emphasize the need to mobilize services for them.[18]

Services for pregnant and postpartum women should include alcohol and/or drug treatment, health care services, and supportive services to assist them in becoming alcohol- or drug-free. Drug treatment services must be offered in different forms to meet individual needs: outpatient services, in-home support, residential treatment, and after-care services. Women who do not receive drug treatment services, family planning, or social services are not only at greater risk for negative health consequences for themselves and their children, but are also at greater risk for repeated drug-exposed births.[19] Prevention, intervention, and after-care services are essential to break the cycle of addiction or abuse and its consequences.

Chemically Exposed Infants and Children

A full array of physical and mental health care services must be available and accessible to infants and children who were exposed prenatally to alcohol or other drugs and who are served by the child welfare system.

The increased use of alcohol and other drugs by pregnant women has resulted in a growing number of infants and children who suffer the effects of prenatal exposure to alcohol or other drugs. According to recent estimates, the number of newborns prenatally exposed to illegal drugs is 554,000 to 739,000 each year.[20] As many as 100,000 cocaine-exposed infants are born each year, and it is projected that by the year 2000, four million children will have been exposed to cocaine prenatally.[21] Fetal Alcohol Syndrome (FAS) affects one in 600 to 750 children; the rate of Fetal Alcohol Effects (FAE) is about twice that of FAS.[22] Where alcoholism has reached epidemic proportions, such as on certain Native American reservations, rates of FAS have been as high as one in 99 births and rates of FAE as high as one in 49 births.[23] Infants and children exposed prenatally to alcohol and other drugs are likely to experience physical, psychological, and developmental problems. They are at heightened risk for low birth weight, premature birth, Sudden Infant Death Syndrome (SIDS), neurological impairment, and developmental and physical disabilities, and they are more likely to suffer from health problems early in life and to die in infancy.[24]

Compounding the adverse effects of initial alcohol or drug exposure in utero, children born to chemically dependent parents may not have the postnatal environment they need to develop and thrive. Chemically dependent parents often face the effects of poverty, unemployment, homelessness, and inadequate health care. Personal and social stresses of parents, combined with a lack of resources, may mean inadequate shelter, improper nutrition, and little health care or nurturance for the children. Difficulties in meeting a child's basic needs may precipitate abusive or neglectful behavior, placing the alcohol- or drug-exposed child at heightened risk of physical, emotional, and developmental problems.

Chemically Involved Youths

A full array of alcohol or other drug abuse prevention and treatment services, including education, alcohol and other drug prevention and counseling, treatment, rehabilitation and after-care services, must be available and accessible to the youths served by the child welfare system.

Developmental changes during adolescence are often accompanied by experimentation with alcohol and other drugs. Alcohol and drugs play a significant role in adolescent injury, accidents, early and unprotected sex, academic underachievement, school dropout rates, poor interpersonal relationships, and psychological problems.[25] Use of alcohol and other drugs can adversely affect a youngster physically, emotionally, and psychologically, and may lead to serious health problems, depression, and suicide. Studies show that 25 percent of adolescents engage in alcohol- and drug- related behaviors that compromise their safety and health,[26] but fewer than one in eight adolescents who need alcohol or other drug treatment actually receive it.[27]

Statistical information on chemical dependency among youths in the child welfare system is virtually nonexistent. A study by Westat, Inc., however, gives one measure of the problem: 17 percent of the youth discharged from out-of-home care between January 1987 and July 1989 reported drug problems and 12 percent reported alcohol problems.[28]

Alcohol. Alcohol is a highly popular substance among teens. A recent report by the U.S. Surgeon General revealed that of the country's 20.7 million teens in 7th through 12th grade, eight million drink alcohol weekly and 454,000 reported that they have five or more drinks consecutively at least once a week.[29] Studies also find that alcohol use begins early: the average age of first use of alcohol is 13.[30] Other studies show that by the senior year of high school, five percent of teens report that they are using alcohol on a daily basis, and 92 percent claim to have tried alcohol at least once.[31]

Adolescent use and abuse of alcohol correlates with serious problems, including driving while alcohol impaired, the major cause of death among teens.[32] Among youth ages 15 to 20, approximately 12 adolescents are killed each day in a drinking and driving incident.[33] Alcohol use is also associated with engaging in unprotected sexual activity; impaired cognitive and physical functioning; impaired health, including liver functioning problems and blood alcohol poisoning; academic failure; depression; and suicide. Importantly, alcohol use also correlates with drug use. Teens who use alcohol are ten times more likely than nondrinkers to use marijuana and 11 times more likely to use cocaine.[34]

Drugs. Drug use among teenagers has declined slightly over the past decade, but adolescents continue to experiment with marijuana, cocaine, crack and other chemical substances.[35] Some adolescents use or experiment with drugs casually while others progress to "problem" drinking, alcoholism, drug abuse, and addiction. Youths who use drugs often engage in other high-risk behaviors simultaneously, including alcohol use, cigarette smoking, and unprotected sex. When drug use is intravenous, the risk of becoming infected with HIV further increases because the virus can be transmitted through the use of a contaminated needle.

Drug use plays an important role in the problems facing the most vulnerable youths. Almost 50 percent of suicidal teenagers used drugs or alcohol close to the time of their deaths, and a significant number of runaways have been or presently are using drugs.[36] Homeless, runaway, throwaway, and gay and lesbian youths are particularly vulnerable to drug abuse and its consequences, including physical health complications, psychological problems, and educational failure.[37]

Marijuana is the most popular illegal drug with teens.[38] In 1991, the National Household Survey on Drug Abuse found that 13 percent of all 12- to 17-year-olds reported having ever used marijuana; 10.1 percent had used it in the past year; and 4.3 percent had used it in the past month.[39] Studies of high school seniors in 1990 showed that 41 percent had tried marijuana in their lifetime, 27 percent reported use in the past year, and 14 percent reported some use in the past month.[40] Adolescents, however, also are involved with other drugs such as cocaine, crack, hallucinogens, sedatives and tranquilizers. The 1990 high school senior study indicated that 18 percent has used stimulants and inhalants; 10 percent had used hallucinogens at least once; 9 percent had used cocaine; and 7 percent had used tranquilizers.[41]

The use of marijuana, cocaine, or other drugs is associated with low self-esteem, poor academic achievement and school attendance, depression, delinquency, use of other substances, and dropping out of school.[42] Adolescents who use drugs are three times more likely to attempt suicide and are more likely to engage in high-risk behaviors that place them at risk for pregnancy, participation in violent crimes, and sexually transmitted diseases, particularly AIDS.[43] Experimentation with and use of drugs is generally linked to parental patterns of alcohol or drug abuse, poor interpersonal and family relationships, neighborhoods in which there is drug activity, and a peer group involved with such activities.[44]

Criminal Activity. Adolescents who abuse alcohol or other drugs have a greater likelihood of involvement in criminal activities and violent behavior relating to drug use. Responses gathered in a study in which teens who used drugs reported on violent events in their lives showed that those teens who use drugs had participated in violent acts more frequently than those who did not use drugs.[45] Violence, injury, and homicide are often related to alcohol and drug use. Studies have found that violence is responsible for as many as 75 percent of all adolescent deaths.[46]

Support Services and Coordination

Health care services must be supported and enhanced by support services for families of the children and youths served by the child welfare system.

Not only do families served by the child welfare system often lack the financial resources to purchase the health care services their children need, they also frequently lack the social supports necessary to use existing resources. The ability of parents to care for their children may be compromised by a number of factors: alcohol or drug abuse by one or more family members; dangerous living conditions due to neighborhood violence and other environmental factors, such as substandard housing and the presence of asbestos or lead; HIV infection or other serious illness affecting one or more family members; and stress unrelieved by child day care services, respite care, and other supportive services. Family vulnerabilities that lead to the involvement of the child welfare system are often related to stresses with health implications. Strains upon the family can escalate to such an extent that children are placed at imminent risk of harm, and the decision must be made to separate the child from the family in order to assure the child's safety.

Before any child is separated from his or her family, supportive services and resources to strengthen the parent's ability to care for the child must be made available. Often times, separation of the child from the family can be avoided through services that enhance family strengths, improve a parent's ability to care for the child, and provide information about and access to available resources, including health care services. Physical and mental health services for parents and/or their children may be essential to resolve the problems confronting the family. Family preservation and support programs that incorporate health care services can strengthen a family at risk of disruption and avert the need to separate children from their parents. Family preservation specialists are finding that families are most likely to benefit from community-based services that offer health care services, as well as supportive services such as child day care, education and counseling services, job training, and services to meet the families' financial and housing needs.

Coordination of Services for Abused or Neglected Children

Coordination between the health care system and the child welfare system must be in place to ensure that the special needs of children and young people who have been abused or neglected are met.

Children and young people served by the child welfare system—in their own homes and in out-of-home care—often have experienced mental and physical injury as a result of physical abuse, sexual abuse and exploitation, negligent treatment, or maltreatment, jeopardizing or undermining their health and well-being.[37] The physical, emotional, and psychological implications of abuse or neglect may be serious and far-reaching, and must be addressed in a comprehensive and coordinated manner. The child welfare and health care systems must collaborate to ensure a timely and effective response to the acute and chronic health problems, mental health difficulties, and developmental problems of children and young people, which often manifest themselves in poor academic achievement and difficulties in interpersonal relationships.

Children and Youths in Their Own Homes. Increasingly, the child welfare system is finding that children and youths served in their own homes are vulnerable youngsters who need a full range of health care services. Of growing concern to child welfare professionals are youngsters who have been exposed to alcohol and other drugs, prenatally or environmentally. Many of these children are receiving child welfare services in their own homes while their families work to resolve the problems that place their children at risk of abuse or neglect. These children may have physiologic, developmental, and cognitive problems that require specialized therapeutic care, in addition to primary health care services. Parents often need assistance in locating and accessing the health care services their children need, and they frequently encounter financial and nonfinancial barriers that prevent access to the necessary services. Coordination and collaboration between the health care and child welfare systems are essential to ensure that children receive the range of needed services.

Children and Youths in Out-of-Home Care. Children and youths are placed in settings such as family foster homes for a number of reasons. Child protective service (CPS) agencies in all states are encountering a growing number of children and youths in need of out-of-home care as a result of abuse and neglect, abandonment, parental alcohol and other drug involvement, the impact of AIDS and HIV on families, and the rising number of infants born to very young mothers who may not be prepared to parent. Since the mid-1980s, the number of children in out-of-home care has risen steadily, from a low of 275,000 in 1983 to approximately 340,000 by end of the 1989.[38] An estimated 442,000 children and youths were in out-of-home care at the end of fiscal year 1992.[39]

Children and youths in out-of-home care are more likely to have physical and emotional problems and developmental and educational difficulties than are other children of comparable age.[40] These children often come from families who have faced a combination of stresses: poverty, unemployment, alcohol and other drug abuse, homelessness, mental illness, and familial violence. Although separation from the family is designed to protect the child, separation can precipitate additional problems for a child. While in out-of-home care, children and youths may experience separation anxiety from siblings and parents, stress associated with adapting to a foster family or other out-of-home care setting, and confusion and guilt associated with separation from their home. The complex array of circumstances associated with being in out-of-home care may have adverse physical, mental, and developmental effects on children. Consequently, children and youths served by the child welfare system outside of their homes are at significant risk for a full range of physical, mental, and developmental problems.

The Need for Coordinated Efforts. Coordination between the health care system and the child welfare system is essential.[41] Health care and child welfare systems must work collaboratively to ensure that the vulnerable children and youths served by the child welfare system receive the health care services they need. Specifically, the health care and child welfare systems must:

- Establish national standards for health care services for children and youths in the child welfare system.

- Create and maintain a medical passport system for each child in out-of-home care to provide an accurate and efficient means of tracking a child's health status and facilitate appropriate health care services and treatment.
- Train caseworkers in the child welfare system regarding the physical, mental health, and developmental needs of children and youths.
- Provide comprehensive screening and treatment for physical, mental health, and development services for children and youths in out-of-home care.

Notes

1 "Health Care Reform: How Do Women, Children and Teens Fare?" Hearing before the Select Committee on Children, Youth and Families, United States House of Representatives, 102nd Congress, 2d Sess., May 5, 1992 (Washington, DC: U.S. Government Printing Office, 1992), p. 5.

2 National Center for Children in Poverty, *Alive and Well? A Research and Policy Review of Health Programs for Poor Young Children* (New York: Columbia University, 1991), p. ix.

3 United States Department of Health and Human Services, Centers for Disease Control, *HIV/AIDS Surveillance Report* 5, 1 (May 1993); *Report of the Presidential Commission on the Human Immunodeficiency Virus Epidemic* (Washington, DC: United States Government Printing Office, 1991)

4 D. Albritten, *Children with HIV/AIDS: A Sourcebook for Caring* (Alexandria, VA: National Association of Children's Hospitals and Related Institutions, 1990).

5 Albritten (1990).

6 J. Laurence, "HIV Infections in Infants and Children," *AIDS Report* (April, 1987): 97-103.

7 Child Welfare League of America, *Meeting the Challenge of HIV Infection in Family Foster Care* (Washington, DC: Child Welfare League of America 1991), pp. 5–13.

8 *HIV/AIDS Surveillance Report* (1993).

9 *HIV/AIDS Surveillance Report* (1993).

10 Centers for Disease Control, HIV/AIDS Surveillance Report 1991.

11 S.B. Manoff, "Acquired Immunodeficiency Syndrome in Adolescents: Epidemiology, Prevention and Public Health Issues," *Current Issues in Pediatrics* 8 (1989): 309–314.

12 S.H. Vermund, K. Hein, H.D. Gayle, J.M. Cary, P.A. Thomas, and E. Drucker, "Acquired Immunodeficiency Syndrome among Adolescents: Case Surveillance Profiles in New York City and the Rest of the United States. *American Journal of Diseases of Children* 143 (1989): 1220–1225.

13 Vermund et al. (1989): 1220–25.

14 National Association of State Alcohol and Drug Abuse Directors (NASADAD), *Treatment Works: A Review of 15 Years of Research Findings* (Washington, DC: NASADAD, 1990), p. 7.

15 NASADAD (1990), p. 7.

16 Operation PAR, "Incidence of Drug Use in Pregnancy in Pinellas County, Florida" (Pinellas County, FL: Juvenile Welfare Board of Pinellas County, October 1989), p. 4.

17 L. Feig, *Drug-Exposed Infants and Children: Service Needs and Policy Questions.* (Washington, DC: U.S. Department of Health and Human Services, August 1990), pp. 4–5; J. Cole, "Legal Intervention during Pregnancy," *Journal of American Medical Association* 264 (November 28, 1990): 36.

18 Feig (1990), p. 5; G. Gittler, "Perinatal Substance Abuse," *Children Today* 19 (July–August 1990): 5.

19 Feig (1990).

20 D.S. Gromby and P. Shiono, "Estimating the Number of Substance Exposed Infants," *The Future of Children: Drug Exposed Infants 1, 1* (Spring 1991): 17–25.

21 R.R. Kusserow, *Crack Babies* (Washington, DC: Office of the Inspector General, OEI-03-89-01540, February 1990), p. 3.

22 A. Streissguth, *Fetal Alcohol Syndrome and the Teratogenicity of Alcohol: Policy Implications* (Prepared for the Eighth World Congress of the International Commission for the Prevention of Alcoholism and Drug Dependency, September 1991), p. 7.

[23] Streissguth (1991).

[24] Feig (1990).

[25] Hechniger (1992), pp. 113-122.

[26] R. MacKenzie, "Substance Abuse," in *The Health of Adolescents,* edited by W. Hendee (San Francisco: Jossey-Bass Publishers, 1991), pp. 186–210.

[27] "Health Care Reform: How Do Women, Children, and Teens Fare?" (1992), p. 5.

[28] Westat, Inc., *A National Evaluation of Title IV-E Foster Care Independent Living Programs for Youth, Final Report,* Phase 1, vol. 1 (Rockville, MD: Westat, Inc., 1991), pp. 4-36.

[29] Hechniger (1992), pp. 714.

[30] C. Carpenter, B. Glassner, B. Johnson, and J. Loughlin, *Kids, Drugs and Crime* (Lexington, MA: Lexington Books, 1988), p. 11.

[31] J.G. Bachman; L.D. Johnson; and P.M. O'Malley, *Monitoring the Future: Questionnaire Responses from the Nation's High School Seniors, 1986* (Ann Arbor: University of Michigan, 1986).

[32] National Commission Against Drunk Driving. *Youth Driving without Impairment. A Community Challenge.* Report on the Youth Impaired Driving Public Hearings (Washington, DC: National Highway Traffic Safety Administration. 1990).

[33] National Commission Against Drunk Driving (1990).

[34] J. Gans, AMA Profiles of Adolescent Health, *America's Adolescents: How Healthy Are They?,* vol. 1 (Chicago: American Medical Association, 1990).

[35] U.S. Department of Health and Human Services, *National Household Survey on Drug Abuse: Population Estimates* (Washington, DC: U.S. Government Printing Office, 1991).

[36] Carpenter (1988), p. 90.

[37] National Network of Runaway and Youth Services, *Substance Abuse and Homeless, Runaway and At Risk Youth* (Washington, DC: National Network of Runaway and Youth Services, 1990).

[38] NIDA (1989).

[39] U.S. Department of Health and Human Services, Public Health Services, National Institute on Drug Abuse (NIDA), *Highlights of the 1991 National*

Household Survey on Drug Abuse (Washington, DC: U.S. Government Printing Office, February 1993).

40 L.D. Johnston, P.M. O'Malley, and J.C. Bachman, *Drug Use Among American High School Seniors, College Students and Young Adults, 1975-1990* (Rockville, MD: National Institute on Drug Abuse, 1991).

41 Johnston et al. (1991).

42 B.S. Mensch and D.B. Kandel, "Dropping Out of School and Drug Involvement," *Sociology of Education* 61 (1988): 95–113.

43 MacKenzie (1991).

44 Carpenter (1988), pp. 11–12.

45 Carpenter (1988), p. 90.

46 Carpenter (1988), pp. 186-193; Hechniger (1992), p. 140.

Beyond The Benefit Package: Overcoming Barriers To Health Care

Certain barriers must be overcome to assure that vulnerable children and youths receive the health care services they need. These barriers must be considered from a financial and structural perspective. Unless they are addressed, the benefit package described in Parts One and Two will not be sufficient, in and of itself, to meet the needs of vulnerable children and youths.

Because of financial barriers to health care, children and youths served by the child welfare system, many of whom live near or below the poverty line, often do not receive quality and appropriate health care. Many of these children and youths are covered by Medicaid and are eligible for health screening and follow-up services through such programs as Medicaid's Early and Periodic Screening, Diagnosis, and Treatment (EPSDT) program or through Head Start. The extent to which these programs meet health needs, however, varies widely, often depending on the degree to which a state has aggressively moved forward in implementing the programs. For many other children, little or no health care is available because of lack of health insurance or, when health insurance coverage is available, because the combination of deductibles, premiums, and copayments creates an insurmountable financial obstacle.

Many children and youths and their families find that the nonfinancial barriers to health care are as difficult to overcome as the financial barriers. Geographic and social isolation, lack of transportation, lack of child day care, cultural barriers, and communication and language difficulties create huge obstacles. Financial barriers and institutional practices, including such factors as service location and office hours, have been cited in at least 15 different studies as two of the major reasons that individuals are unable to obtain sufficient health care.[1] The health care system must be designed to ensure that health care services are not only available, but are accessible to vulnerable children and youths.

FINANCIAL BARRIERS TO ACCESS

Primary and specialized health care services must be available without cost-sharing requirements to pregnant women and to the children and youths served by the child welfare system.

Currently, health care insurance is tied largely to employment and is offered as an employment benefit at a cost more affordable than individual purchase of coverage might be. The extent to which employers provide health insurance, however, has begun to decline as health care costs have escalated.[2] During the past decade, the proportion of employers who paid 100 percent of the annual premium for family coverage declined from 51 percent to 23 percent.[3] At the same time, a growing number of employers do not offer health insurance as an employment benefit, and workers and their families are forced to obtain health care coverage through another means or to forego coverage. Children are most likely to be uninsured, particularly if their parents work for a business with fewer than 25 employees or are self-employed.[4] For some families who do not have employment-based health coverage, health insurance is provided by Medicaid. Working, two-parent families, however, are unlikely to qualify for the Medicaid program. In many instances, they do not meet the specific age, disability, family structure or income requirements to qualify for the program. As a result, significant numbers of low-income children, youths, and pregnant women find themselves in a health care predicament: their employers do not offer health insurance, or they are unemployed and are ineligible for Medicaid.

Simply extending health insurance coverage as presently designed, however, is not sufficient. Even if health insurance in its present form were extended to children, youths, and pregnant women, financial access to needed health care services would not be guaranteed because of the current system's required copayments in the form of premiums, deductibles, and partial payments for services. Under many health insurance policies, for example, mental health services are treated as a specialty service and are subject to a copayment. A family whose child needs intensive mental health services for an extended period of time may well find the required copayment to be prohibitive. Similarly, many preventive services are omitted from primary care benefits packages because of the costs associated with those services. Families may find it impossible to access such services because of the costs.

Families served by the child welfare system tend to have incomes at or below the poverty level and, as a result, are likely to encounter significant financial barriers to health care. These families, however, are most at risk for physical, mental health, and developmental problems and are most in need of primary, preventive, and specialized health care services. For these families, cost-sharing requirements pose a significant barrier to health care access. At a minimum, cost sharing must be eliminated for the children, youths, and pregnant women served by the child welfare system.

Nonfinancial Barriers to Access

Nonfinancial barriers to health care, including institutional practices, transportation, limited availability of providers, cultural and language barriers, and poor service coordination, must be recognized and addressed.

Even if families have health insurance that gives them financial access to health care without cost-sharing requirements, accessibility remains a problem because of other barriers. A recent study, for example, discovered that pregnant women with Medicaid coverage are less likely to receive adequate prenatal care than women with no insurance at all.[5] Medicaid recipients in that study reported substantial barriers to prenatal care in the form of inconveniently located health care facilities, no consistent source of health care, and absence of child day care resources.[6] Other factors also substantially affect access to health care services: institutional practices such as inconvenient service hours, service fragmentation in terms of the location of services, lengthy and demeaning application procedures, lack of transportation, the absence of a sufficient number of physicians and health care providers in rural areas and inner cities, an insufficient number of specialty service providers, and language and cultural barriers.

Inconvenient Office Hours and Lack of Child Day Care

Inconvenient office and clinic hours may pose significant problems for families. In one study, for example, women who received inadequate prenatal care cited an inability to arrange time off from work as a major difficulty.[7] These problems are accentuated when parents work or when dependence on public transportation limits flexibility in scheduling appointments. Likewise, a parent, particularly a sole caregiver, may be unable to seek health care for one child without day care services for other children. In one survey concerning failure to obtain prenatal care, almost one-quarter of obstetricians and 16 percent of women reported that the absence of child care posed a significant obstacle to obtaining health care.[8]

Transportation

Transportation problems frequently pose a significant barrier to health care. Many families who need health care for their children do not have a car or lack money for bus or taxi fares, and facilities may not be in walking distance. In one study, 23 percent of women who received inadequate prenatal care and 38 percent of their physicians cited transportation difficulties as an important factor in keeping them from receiving care.[9]

Insufficient Numbers of Providers

Many families do not receive care because they live in medically underserved areas or geographically isolated communities that lack a sufficient number of health care providers and facilities. More than 33 million Americans live in areas that have been federally designated as health professional shortage areas.[10] More than three-quarters of the medically underserved live in urban areas; rural counties, however, are 2.8 times more likely to be medically underserved than urban counties.[11] Studies reveal that obstetrical services in particular are often unavailable. One study found that approximately 215,000 births occur each year in 799 counties that lack any clinic provider.[12] Another study found that each year 110,000 women give birth in counties that have no office-based obstetrician-gynecologist or clinic that provides prenatal care.[13] Access to providers also may be limited because of provider unwillingness to participate in government funded health care programs such as Medicaid.[14] Between 1987 and 1989, for example, the percentage of pediatricians who accepted Medicaid patients decreased from 85 percent to 77 percent.[15]

Language and Cultural Concerns

Language and cultural barriers pose challenges to service providers and patients. Health care providers must be prepared to address cultural concerns, perspectives, and practices if health care is to be meaningfully provided. This process is facilitated when health care providers are representative of the cultural and ethnic groups they serve. Language and communication differences may also pose a substantial barrier. Health care workers who are bilingual, who understand cultural differences, and who are trained in communication with the hearing-impaired can avoid miscommunication and can assist parents in utilizing existing health care services for their children.

Poor Coordination of Services

Families often need a variety of health and social services. When there is no coordination of services, they may be able to meet their needs only by going to multiple locations and completing multiple application forms. Resources often needed by families such as Aid to Families with Dependent Children (AFDC), Medicaid, Food Stamps, Head Start, and the Supplemental Food Program for Women, Infants and Children (WIC) are administered by different federal agencies and often are implemented by different state agencies or departments. Although the programs serve many of the same clients, they frequently operate under different service definitions and eligibility requirements, lack the ability to coordinate the services and resources of one another, and confuse families with contradictory information and fragmented approaches to services.

Community-based centers can offer single locations for health care and social services for neighborhoods. Such centers can maximize access because of their proximity to the clients they serve, the likelihood that clients will feel more comfortable in a familiar environment, convenient service hours, and coordination of multiple services in a "one-stop" shopping environment. Community-based centers, whether in a school or in another facility, can provide a range of services that families need: drug prevention services, prenatal care, primary pediatric care, immunizations, WIC, Food Stamps, and transportation services. Coordination may be enhanced as well through the use of shortened or joint application forms, outreach programs, formal or informal interagency cooperation agreements, and training of health care and other service providers regarding the language and cultural practices of the communities they serve.

NOTES

1 Institute of Medicine, 1988.

2 The Mildred and Claude Pepper Foundation, "Financing National Health Care: A Nationwide Survey of Voters' Opinions" (May 15, 1992).

3 "Health Care Reform: How Do Women, Children and Teens Fare?" Hearing before the Select Committee on Children, Youth and Families, United States House of Representatives, 102nd Congress, 2d Sess., May 5, 1992 (Washington, DC: U.S. Government Printing Office, 1992), p. 4.

4 "Health Care Reform: How Do Women, Children and Teens Fare?" (1992), p. 4.

5 "Pregnant Medicaid Recipients Get Less Care Than Uninsured," *Youth Law News* [November–December 1991]: 5

6 *Youth Law News* (1991): 5

7 "Health Care Reform: How Do Women, Children and Teens Fare?" (1992), p. 8.

8 "Generating Innovative Strategies for Healthy Infants and Children," Hearing Before the Select Committee on Children, Youth and Families, House of Representatives, 102nd Congress, 1st Session, April 23, 1991 (Washington, DC: U.S. Government Printing Office, 1991), p. 7.

9 Generating Innovative Strategies (1991), p. 8.

10 "Health Care Reform: How Do Women, Children and Teens Fare?" (1992), p. 7.

11 "Health Care Reform: How Do Women, Children and Teen Fare?" (1992), p. 6.

12 Generating Innovative Strategies (1991), p. 8.

13 Generating Innovative Strategies (1991), p. 8.

14 Generating Innovative Strategies (1991), p. 7.

15 "Health Care Reform: How Do Women, Children and Teens Fare?" (1992), p. 7.

CONCLUSION

The health care system, urgently in need of reform, must address the needs of the vulnerable children and youths served by the child welfare system. These youngsters, having experienced abuse, neglect, and abandonment, are at particular risk of physical health, mental health, and developmental problems. Under the current health care system, however, they are among those least likely to receive the services they need. Primary health care services must be available to pregnant women and the infants, toddlers, school-age children and adolescents served by the child welfare system. Support services and specialized health care services, services relating to HIV and AIDS, and alcohol and other drug abuse prevention and treatment services must also be available. Finally, these services must be offered to pregnant women and the children and youths served by the child welfare system with no cost-sharing requirements and with attention to the nonfinancial barriers to access to health care. With a true commitment to health care reform, the most vulnerable children and youths in America will receive the full range of health services they so urgently need.